HIGH PROTEIN VEGAN MEALS FOR TYPE 2 DIABETICS

Delicious Plant-Based Recipes for Blood Sugar Management & Balanced Nutrition

By Mia Bennett

COPYRIGHT PAGE

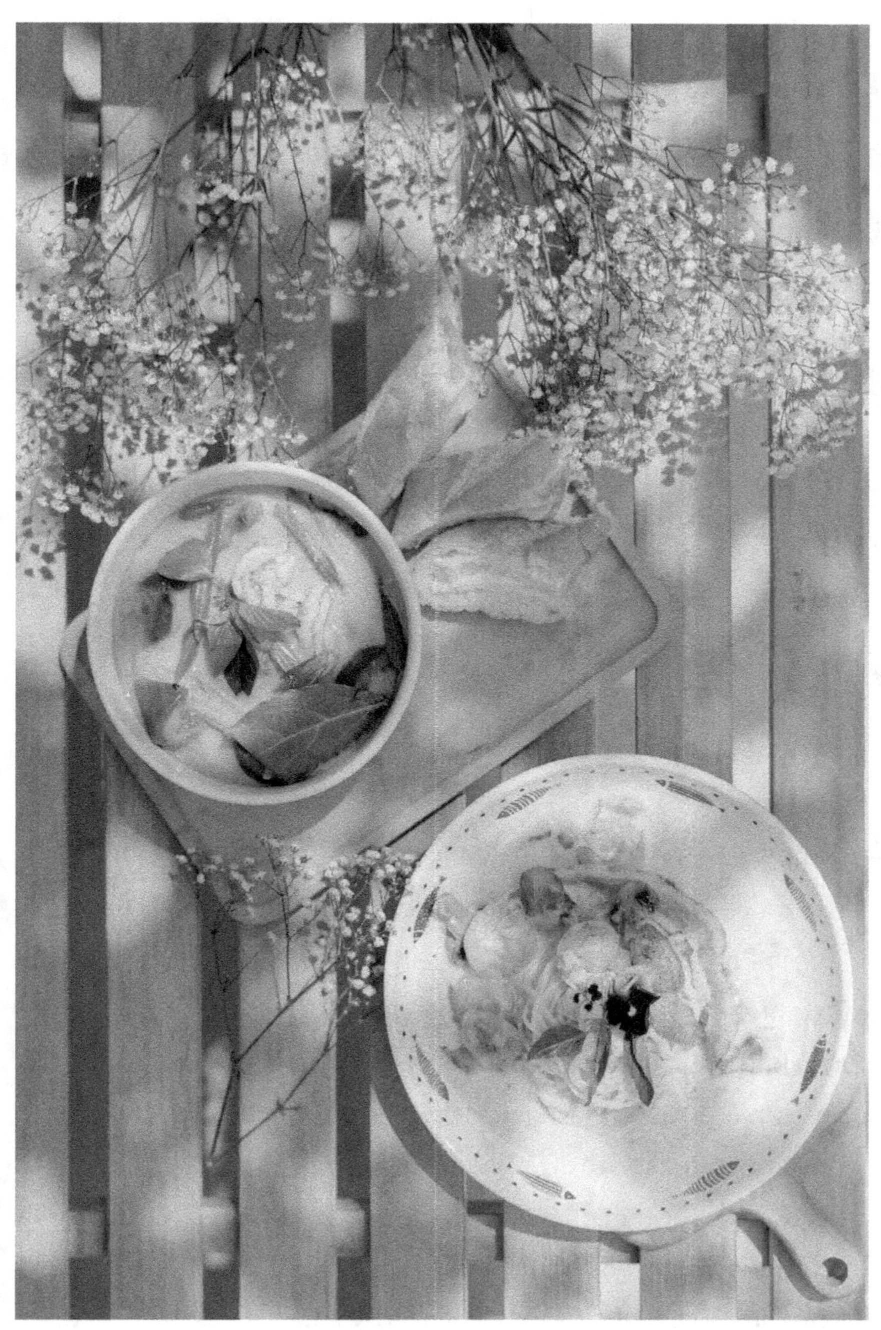

TABLE OF CONTENTS

Chapter 3: Lunch Recipes.. 38

Chapter 4: Dinner Recipes 58

Chapter 5: Snacks and Appetizers 78

Chapter 6: Desserts 94

Chapter 7: Smoothies 116

INTRODUCTION

I magine your body is a grand estate, and insulin is the key that unlocks the gates to your cells, allowing sugar (glucose) to enter and fuel them. In Type 2 Diabetes, this system gets a bit jammed. Either your body doesn't produce enough insulin, or the cells become resistant to its message. This sugar backup in the bloodstream can lead to a cascade of health problems.

The Potential of a High-Protein Vegan Diet:

Here's where a well-planned high-protein vegan diet enters the scene. Unlike traditional diabetic diets that often focus on restricting carbohydrates, a plant-based approach with ample protein offers a unique set of benefits:

- **Weight Management**: Many people with Type 2 Diabetes struggle with weight management. Vegan diets tend to be naturally lower in calories and fat, promoting healthy weight loss.
- **Blood Sugar Control:** Studies suggest that plant-based proteins like lentils, beans, and tofu may help regulate blood

sugar levels by inducing a slower, steadier rise in glucose compared to animal proteins.

- **Fiber Powerhouse:** Vegan meals are bursting with fiber, which slows down digestion and sugar absorption, further aiding blood sugar control.
- **Heart-Healthy Benefits**: A plant-based diet is typically lower in saturated fat and cholesterol, promoting heart health, a critical concern for those with diabetes.

Nutritional Considerations for Success:

While vegan diets offer a treasure trove of nutrients, there are a few key players to keep on your radar for optimal diabetic management:

- **Protein**: Aim for a variety of plant-based protein sources throughout the day, like tofu, tempeh, lentils, beans, nuts, and seeds.
- **Healthy Fats:** Include good fats like those found in avocados, olives, nuts, and seeds to promote satiety and nutrient absorption.
- **Micronutrients**: Be mindful of getting enough vitamin B12, essential for nerve health, which can be lower in vegan diets. Fortified foods or supplements can help bridge the gap.

Planning and Prepping Your Vegan Feast:

Meal planning is your secret weapon for a successful vegan journey with diabetes. Here are some tips:

- **Batch Cooking**: Dedicate some time each week to cook a big pot of lentil soup, a veggie chili, or a hearty tofu stir-fry. These become lifesavers for busy days.
- **Stock Up on Staples:** Keep your pantry stocked with dry beans, lentils, brown rice, quinoa, and frozen vegetables for quick and healthy meals.
- **Snack Smart:** Have a stash of grab-and-go snacks like nuts, seeds, veggie sticks with hummus, or sliced fruit with a nut butter drizzle.
- **Spice Up Your Life:** Experiment with herbs and spices to add flavor and variety to your meals, keeping things interesting.

Remember: With a little planning and creativity, you can unlock a world of delicious and nutritious vegan meals that empower you to manage your Type 2 Diabetes effectively.

Chapter 1: 30 Day Meal Plan

Week 1

Day 1

- Breakfast: Tofu Scramble with Spinach and Mushrooms
- Lunch: Chickpea Salad Sandwich
- Dinner: Lentil Shepherd's Pie
- Snack: Roasted Chickpeas
- Dessert: Chia Seed Pudding with Coconut Milk

Day 2

- Breakfast: Chia Seed Pudding with Berries
- Lunch: Quinoa and Black Bean Salad
- Dinner: Vegan Stuffed Bell Peppers
- Snack: Veggie Sticks with Hummus
- Dessert: Vegan Protein Brownies

Day 3

- Breakfast: Quinoa Breakfast Bowl with Almonds and Coconut
- Lunch: Vegan Buddha Bowl with Tahini Dressing
- Dinner: Chickpea and Sweet Potato Curry
- Snack: Spicy Edamame

- Dessert: Almond Butter and Dark Chocolate Energy Balls

Day 4

- Breakfast: Avocado Toast with Hemp Seeds
- Lunch: Lentil Soup with Spinach
- Dinner: Tofu and Broccoli Stir-Fry
- Snack: Vegan Stuffed Mushrooms
- Dessert: Baked Apple Slices with Cinnamon

Day 5

- Breakfast: Vegan Protein Pancakes with Fresh Berries
- Lunch: Tofu and Vegetable Stir-Fry
- Dinner: Vegan Black Bean Burgers
- Snack: Almond Flour Crackers with Guacamole
- Dessert: Vegan Chocolate Avocado Mousse

Day 6

- Breakfast: Overnight Oats with Almond Butter and Chia Seeds
- Lunch: Spicy Chickpea Wraps
- Dinner: Eggplant and Chickpea Stew
- Snack: Baked Tofu Bites
- Dessert: Coconut and Almond Flour Cookies

Day 7

- Breakfast: Breakfast Burrito with Black Beans and Tofu
- Lunch: Vegan Caesar Salad with Crispy Chickpeas
- Dinner: Quinoa-Stuffed Acorn Squash
- Snack: Kale Chips
- Dessert: Berry Crumble with Oat Topping

Week 2

Day 8

- Breakfast: Smoothie Bowl with Mixed Berries and Pumpkin Seeds
- Lunch: Lentil and Vegetable Stuffed Peppers
- Dinner: Vegan Chili with Lentils and Beans
- Snack: Lentil and Veggie Spring Rolls
- Dessert: Vegan Banana Bread

Day 9

- Breakfast: Vegan Breakfast Sausage Patties
- Lunch: Edamame and Quinoa Salad
- Dinner: Grilled Portobello Mushrooms with Quinoa
- Snack: Vegan Cheese Dip with Crudités
- Dessert: Chocolate Chia Seed Pudding

Day 10

- Breakfast: Lentil and Vegetable Breakfast Hash
- Lunch: Vegan Sushi Rolls with Brown Rice
- Dinner: Thai Peanut Tofu and Vegetable Noodles
- Snack: Stuffed Mini Peppers with Hummus
- Dessert: Raw Vegan Cheesecake

Day 11

- Breakfast: Vegan Omelette with Chickpea Flour
- Lunch: Chickpea and Spinach Curry
- Dinner: Spaghetti with Lentil Bolognese
- Snack: Zucchini Fritters
- Dessert: Mango Sorbet

Day 12

- Breakfast: Almond Flour Muffins with Blueberries
- Lunch: Grilled Vegetable and Quinoa Salad
- Dinner: Baked Tempeh with Vegetables
- Snack: Spicy Roasted Cauliflower
- Dessert: Vegan Carrot Cake

Day 13

- Breakfast: Green Smoothie with Spinach and Protein Powder

- Lunch: Spaghetti Squash with Lentil Marinara
- Dinner: Vegan Paella with Chickpeas and Vegetables
- Snack: Vegan Spinach Artichoke Dip
- Dessert: Peanut Butter and Chocolate Smoothie Bowl

Day 14

- Breakfast: Buckwheat Porridge with Nuts and Seeds
- Lunch: Zucchini Noodles with Avocado Pesto
- Dinner: Stuffed Zucchini Boats with Quinoa
- Snack: Avocado and Black Bean Salsa
- Dessert: Vegan Lemon Bars

Week 3

Day 15

- Breakfast: Sweet Potato and Black Bean Breakfast Bowl
- Lunch: Roasted Chickpea and Vegetable Bowl
- Dinner: Cauliflower and Chickpea Tacos
- Snack: Sweet Potato Bites with Avocado
- Dessert: Cinnamon Roasted Chickpeas

Day 16

- Breakfast: Tofu Scramble with Spinach and Mushrooms
- Lunch: Chickpea Salad Sandwich

- Dinner: Lentil Shepherd's Pie
- Snack: Roasted Chickpeas
- Dessert: Chia Seed Pudding with Coconut Milk

Day 17

- Breakfast: Chia Seed Pudding with Berries
- Lunch: Quinoa and Black Bean Salad
- Dinner: Vegan Stuffed Bell Peppers
- Snack: Veggie Sticks with Hummus
- Dessert: Vegan Protein Brownies

Day 18

- Breakfast: Quinoa Breakfast Bowl with Almonds and Coconut
- Lunch: Vegan Buddha Bowl with Tahini Dressing
- Dinner: Chickpea and Sweet Potato Curry
- Snack: Spicy Edamame
- Dessert: Almond Butter and Dark Chocolate Energy Balls

Day 19

- Breakfast: Avocado Toast with Hemp Seeds
- Lunch: Lentil Soup with Spinach
- Dinner: Tofu and Broccoli Stir-Fry
- Snack: Vegan Stuffed Mushrooms

- Dessert: Baked Apple Slices with Cinnamon

Day 20

- Breakfast: Vegan Protein Pancakes with Fresh Berries
- Lunch: Tofu and Vegetable Stir-Fry
- Dinner: Vegan Black Bean Burgers
- Snack: Almond Flour Crackers with Guacamole
- Dessert: Vegan Chocolate Avocado Mousse

Day 21

- Breakfast: Overnight Oats with Almond Butter and Chia Seeds
- Lunch: Spicy Chickpea Wraps
- Dinner: Eggplant and Chickpea Stew
- Snack: Baked Tofu Bites
- Dessert: Coconut and Almond Flour Cookies

Week 4

Day 22

- Breakfast: Breakfast Burrito with Black Beans and Tofu
- Lunch: Vegan Caesar Salad with Crispy Chickpeas
- Dinner: Quinoa-Stuffed Acorn Squash
- Snack: Kale Chips

- Dessert: Berry Crumble with Oat Topping

Day 23

- Breakfast: Smoothie Bowl with Mixed Berries and Pumpkin Seeds
- Lunch: Lentil and Vegetable Stuffed Peppers
- Dinner: Vegan Chili with Lentils and Beans
- Snack: Lentil and Veggie Spring Rolls
- Dessert: Vegan Banana Bread

Day 24

- Breakfast: Vegan Breakfast Sausage Patties
- Lunch: Edamame and Quinoa Salad
- Dinner: Grilled Portobello Mushrooms with Quinoa
- Snack: Vegan Cheese Dip with Crudités
- Dessert: Chocolate Chia Seed Pudding

Day 25

- Breakfast: Lentil and Vegetable Breakfast Hash
- Lunch: Vegan Sushi Rolls with Brown Rice
- Dinner: Thai Peanut Tofu and Vegetable Noodles
- Snack: Stuffed Mini Peppers with Hummus
- Dessert: Raw Vegan Cheesecake

Day 26

- Breakfast: Vegan Omelette with Chickpea Flour
- Lunch: Chickpea and Spinach Curry
- Dinner: Spaghetti with Lentil Bolognese
- Snack: Zucchini Fritters
- Dessert: Mango Sorbet

Day 27

- Breakfast: Almond Flour Muffins with Blueberries
- Lunch: Grilled Vegetable and Quinoa Salad
- Dinner: Baked Tempeh with Vegetables
- Snack: Spicy Roasted Cauliflower
- Dessert: Vegan Carrot Cake

Day 28

- Breakfast: Green Smoothie with Spinach and Protein Powder
- Lunch: Spaghetti Squash with Lentil Marinara
- Dinner: Vegan Paella with Chickpeas and Vegetables
- Snack: Vegan Spinach Artichoke Dip
- Dessert: Peanut Butter and Chocolate Smoothie Bowl

Day 29

- Breakfast: Buckwheat Porridge with Nuts and Seeds

- Lunch: Zucchini Noodles with Avocado Pesto
- Dinner: Stuffed Zucchini Boats with Quinoa
- Snack: Avocado and Black Bean Salsa
- Dessert: Vegan Lemon Bars

Day 30

- Breakfast: Sweet Potato and Black Bean Breakfast Bowl
- Lunch: Roasted Chickpea and Vegetable Bowl
- Dinner: Cauliflower and Chickpea Tacos
- Snack: Sweet Potato Bites with Avocado
- Dessert: Cinnamon Roasted Chickpeas

Chapter 2: Breakfast Recipes

A wholesome breakfast sets the tone for the day, especially for individuals managing type 2 diabetes. The following high-protein vegan breakfast recipes are designed to provide sustained energy, balance blood sugar levels, and keep you full longer.

Tofu Scramble with Spinach and Mushrooms

Ingredients:

- 1 block firm tofu, crumbled
- 1 cup spinach, chopped
- 1 cup mushrooms, sliced
- 1 small onion, diced
- 1 clove garlic, minced
- 1 tbsp olive oil
- 1 tsp turmeric
- Salt and pepper to taste

Instructions:

1. Heat olive oil in a pan over medium heat.
2. Sauté onion and garlic until fragrant.
3. Add mushrooms and cook until tender.

4. Stir in tofu, spinach, and turmeric. Cook for 5-7 minutes.

5. Season with salt and pepper.

Nutrition Information (per serving):

- Calories: 200
- Protein: 15g
- Carbohydrates: 10g
- Fat: 12g
- Fiber: 4g
- Sugar: 2g
- Portion size: 1 cup

Chia Seed Pudding with Berries

Ingredients:

- 1/4 cup chia seeds
- 1 cup almond milk
- 1 tsp vanilla extract
- 1 tbsp maple syrup
- 1/2 cup mixed berries

Instructions:

1. Mix chia seeds, almond milk, vanilla, and maple syrup in a bowl.

2. Refrigerate overnight.

3. Top with mixed berries before serving.

Nutrition Information (per serving):

- Calories: 250
- Protein: 6g
- Carbohydrates: 30g
- Fat: 12g
- Fiber: 10g
- Sugar: 12g
- Portion size: 1 cup

Quinoa Breakfast Bowl with Almonds and Coconut

Ingredients:

- 1/2 cup quinoa, cooked
- 1/4 cup almonds, chopped
- 1/4 cup shredded coconut
- 1 tbsp maple syrup
- 1/2 tsp cinnamon

Instructions:

1. Combine cooked quinoa, almonds, coconut, and cinnamon in a bowl.
2. Drizzle with maple syrup and serve.

Nutrition Information (per serving):

- Calories: 300
- Protein: 8g
- Carbohydrates: 35g
- Fat: 15g
- Fiber: 6g
- Sugar: 10g
- Portion size: 1 bowl

Avocado Toast with Hemp Seeds

Ingredients:

- 1 ripe avocado
- 2 slices whole grain bread
- 1 tbsp hemp seeds
- Salt and pepper to taste
- Red pepper flakes (optional)

Instructions:

1. Toast the bread slices.

2. Mash the avocado and spread evenly on the toast.

3. Sprinkle with hemp seeds, salt, pepper, and red pepper flakes if desired.

Nutrition Information (per serving):

- Calories: 300
- Protein: 8g
- Carbohydrates: 32g
- Fat: 18g
- Fiber: 10g
- Sugar: 2g
- Portion size: 2 slices

Vegan Protein Pancakes with Fresh Berries

Ingredients:

- 1 cup whole wheat flour
- 1 scoop vegan protein powder
- 1 tbsp baking powder
- 1 tbsp flaxseed meal
- 1 cup almond milk

- 1 tbsp maple syrup
- 1 cup fresh berries

Instructions:

1. Mix dry ingredients in a bowl.
2. Add almond milk and maple syrup, stirring until smooth.
3. Cook pancakes on a non-stick pan over medium heat.
4. Serve with fresh berries.

Nutrition Information (per serving):

- Calories: 350
- Protein: 12g
- Carbohydrates: 55g
- Fat: 8g
- Fiber: 10g
- Sugar: 15g
- Portion size: 3 pancakes

Overnight Oats with Almond Butter and Chia Seeds

Ingredients:

- 1/2 cup rolled oats
- 1 cup almond milk

- 1 tbsp almond butter
- 1 tbsp chia seeds
- 1 tsp maple syrup

Instructions:

1. Combine oats, almond milk, almond butter, chia seeds, and maple syrup in a jar.
2. Refrigerate overnight.
3. Stir before serving.

Nutrition Information (per serving):

- Calories: 300
- Protein: 10g
- Carbohydrates: 40g
- Fat: 12g
- Fiber: 10g
- Sugar: 8g
- Portion size: 1 jar

Breakfast Burrito with Black Beans and Tofu

Ingredients:

- 1/2 cup black beans, cooked

- 1/2 cup tofu, crumbled
- 1/4 cup salsa
- 1 whole grain tortilla
- 1/4 avocado, sliced

Instructions:

1. Combine black beans, tofu, and salsa in a bowl.
2. Heat mixture in a pan over medium heat.
3. Fill tortilla with the mixture and avocado slices.

Nutrition Information (per serving):

- Calories: 350
- Protein: 15g
- Carbohydrates: 45g
- Fat: 12g
- Fiber: 12g
- Sugar: 4g
- Portion size: 1 burrito

Smoothie Bowl with Mixed Berries and Pumpkin Seeds

Ingredients:

- 1 cup mixed berries

- 1/2 banana
- 1/2 cup almond milk
- 1 tbsp pumpkin seeds
- 1 tbsp shredded coconut

Instructions:

1. Blend berries, banana, and almond milk until smooth.
2. Pour into a bowl and top with pumpkin seeds and shredded coconut.

Nutrition Information (per serving):

- Calories: 250
- Protein: 5g
- Carbohydrates: 40g
- Fat: 8g
- Fiber: 8g
- Sugar: 20g
- Portion size: 1 bowl

Vegan Breakfast Sausage Patties

Ingredients:

- 1 cup lentils, cooked
- 1/2 cup oats

- 1/4 cup walnuts, chopped
- 1 tbsp soy sauce
- 1 tsp sage
- 1 tsp thyme
- Salt and pepper to taste

Instructions:

1. Combine all ingredients in a food processor until well mixed.
2. Form into patties and cook on a non-stick pan until browned on both sides.

Nutrition Information (per serving):

- Calories: 200
- Protein: 10g
- Carbohydrates: 25g
- Fat: 8g
- Fiber: 6g
- Sugar: 2g
- Portion size: 2 patties

Lentil and Vegetable Breakfast Hash

Ingredients:

- 1 cup lentils, cooked

- 1 bell pepper, diced
- 1 small onion, diced
- 1 small zucchini, diced
- 1 tbsp olive oil
- Salt and pepper to taste

Instructions:

1. Heat olive oil in a pan over medium heat.
2. Sauté onion, bell pepper, and zucchini until tender.
3. Add lentils and cook for 5 minutes.
4. Season with salt and pepper.

Nutrition Information (per serving):

- Calories: 250
- Protein: 12g
- Carbohydrates: 35g
- Fat: 8g
- Fiber: 10g
- Sugar: 8g
- Portion size: 1 cup

Vegan Omelette with Chickpea Flour

Ingredients:

- 1/2 cup chickpea flour
- 1/2 cup water
- 1/4 cup spinach, chopped
- 1/4 cup mushrooms, diced
- 1/4 cup bell pepper, diced
- 1 tbsp nutritional yeast
- Salt and pepper to taste

Instructions:

1. Mix chickpea flour and water until smooth.
2. Stir in spinach, mushrooms, bell pepper, nutritional yeast, salt, and pepper.
3. Cook on a non-stick pan over medium heat until set.

Nutrition Information (per serving):

- Calories: 200
- Protein: 10g
- Carbohydrates: 25g
- Fat: 6g
- Fiber: 5g
- Sugar: 3g
- Portion size: 1 omelette

Almond Flour Muffins with Blueberries

Ingredients:

- 2 cups almond flour
- 1 tsp baking powder
- 1/4 cup maple syrup
- 1/4 cup almond milk
- 1 cup blueberries

Instructions:

1. Preheat oven to 350°F (175°C).
2. Mix almond flour, baking powder, maple syrup, and almond milk in a bowl.
3. Fold in blueberries.
4. Divide batter into muffin tins and bake for 20-25 minutes.

Nutrition Information (per serving):

- Calories: 200
- Protein: 6g
- Carbohydrates: 18g
- Fat: 12g
- Fiber: 4g
- Sugar: 10g
- Portion size: 1 muffin

Green Smoothie with Spinach and Protein Powder

Ingredients:

- 1 cup spinach
- 1/2 banana
- 1 cup almond milk
- 1 scoop vegan protein powder
- 1 tbsp flaxseed meal

Instructions:

1. Blend all ingredients until smooth.
2. Serve immediately.

Nutrition Information (per serving):

- Calories: 250
- Protein: 20g
- Carbohydrates: 30g
- Fat: 6g
- Fiber: 6g
- Sugar: 12g
- Portion size: 1 smoothie

Buckwheat Porridge with Nuts and Seeds

Ingredients:

- 1/2 cup buckwheat groats
- 1 cup almond milk
- 1/4 cup mixed nuts and seeds
- 1 tbsp maple syrup
- 1/2 tsp cinnamon

Instructions:

1. Cook buckwheat groats in almond milk until tender.
2. Stir in maple syrup and cinnamon.
3. Top with mixed nuts and seeds.

Nutrition Information (per serving):

- Calories: 300
- Protein: 10g
- Carbohydrates: 45g
- Fat: 12g
- Fiber: 8g
- Sugar: 10g
- Portion size: 1 bowl

Sweet Potato and Black Bean Breakfast Bowl

Ingredients:

- 1 small sweet potato, diced
- 1/2 cup black beans, cooked
- 1/4 avocado, sliced
- 1 tbsp salsa
- 1 tbsp nutritional yeast

Instructions:

1. Roast sweet potato at 400°F (200°C) for 25-30 minutes.
2. Combine roasted sweet potato, black beans, avocado, salsa, and nutritional yeast in a bowl.

Nutrition Information (per serving):

- Calories: 300
- Protein: 10g
- Carbohydrates: 45g
- Fat: 10g
- Fiber: 12g
- Sugar: 10g
- Portion size: 1 bowl

Chapter 3: Lunch Recipes

Eating a well-balanced, high-protein vegan lunch can be both satisfying and beneficial for managing Type 2 diabetes. The following recipes are designed to provide plenty of plant-based protein while keeping carbohydrate levels in check.

Chickpea Salad Sandwich

Ingredients:

- 1 can chickpeas, drained and rinsed
- 2 tbsp vegan mayonnaise
- 1 tbsp Dijon mustard
- 1 stalk celery, chopped
- 1 small red onion, finely chopped
- 1 tbsp lemon juice
- Salt and pepper to taste
- 4 slices whole grain bread
- Lettuce leaves

Instructions:

1. In a bowl, mash the chickpeas with a fork.
2. Add vegan mayonnaise, mustard, celery, red onion, lemon juice, salt, and pepper. Mix well.

3. Spread the mixture on bread slices and top with lettuce leaves.

4. Serve as a sandwich.

Nutrition Information (per sandwich):

- Calories: 290
- Protein: 12g
- Carbohydrates: 40g
- Fat: 8g
- Fiber: 8g
- Sugar: 4g
- Portion size: 1 sandwich

Quinoa and Black Bean Salad

Ingredients:

- 1 cup quinoa, cooked
- 1 can black beans, drained and rinsed
- 1 red bell pepper, chopped
- 1 small red onion, chopped
- 1 cup corn kernels
- 1 avocado, diced
- Juice of 1 lime
- 2 tbsp olive oil

- 1 tsp cumin

- Salt and pepper to taste

Instructions:

1. In a large bowl, combine quinoa, black beans, bell pepper, red onion, corn, and avocado.

2. In a small bowl, whisk together lime juice, olive oil, cumin, salt, and pepper.

3. Pour the dressing over the salad and toss to combine.

Nutrition Information (per serving):

- Calories: 350

- Protein: 12g

- Carbohydrates: 45g

- Fat: 14g

- Fiber: 11g

- Sugar: 3g

- Portion size: 1 cup

Vegan Buddha Bowl with Tahini Dressing

Ingredients:

- 1 cup cooked brown rice

- 1 cup chickpeas, roasted

- 1 cup steamed broccoli
- 1 carrot, shredded
- 1/2 cucumber, sliced
- 1 avocado, sliced
- 2 tbsp tahini
- Juice of 1 lemon
- 1 tbsp maple syrup
- 1 tbsp water
- Salt and pepper to taste

Instructions:

1. In a bowl, arrange brown rice, chickpeas, broccoli, carrot, cucumber, and avocado.
2. In a small bowl, whisk together tahini, lemon juice, maple syrup, water, salt, and pepper.
3. Drizzle the tahini dressing over the Buddha bowl.

Nutrition Information (per bowl):

- Calories: 400
- Protein: 14g
- Carbohydrates: 50g
- Fat: 18g
- Fiber: 12g
- Sugar: 5g

- Portion size: 1 bowl

Lentil Soup with Spinach

Ingredients:

- 1 cup lentils, rinsed
- 1 onion, chopped
- 2 cloves garlic, minced
- 1 carrot, chopped
- 1 celery stalk, chopped
- 6 cups vegetable broth
- 2 cups fresh spinach
- 1 tsp cumin
- 1 tsp thyme
- Salt and pepper to taste

Instructions:

1. In a large pot, sauté onion, garlic, carrot, and celery until softened.
2. Add lentils, vegetable broth, cumin, thyme, salt, and pepper.
3. Bring to a boil, then reduce heat and simmer for 30 minutes.
4. Stir in spinach and cook until wilted.

Nutrition Information (per serving):

- Calories: 180
- Protein: 12g
- Carbohydrates: 30g
- Fat: 2g
- Fiber: 11g
- Sugar: 4g
- Portion size: 1 cup

Tofu and Vegetable Stir-Fry

Ingredients:

- 1 block firm tofu, cubed
- 2 tbsp soy sauce
- 1 tbsp sesame oil
- 1 bell pepper, sliced
- 1 broccoli head, chopped
- 1 carrot, sliced
- 1 zucchini, sliced
- 2 cloves garlic, minced
- 1 tbsp grated ginger
- 1 tbsp olive oil

Instructions:

1. Marinate tofu in soy sauce for 10 minutes.
2. In a pan, heat olive oil and add garlic and ginger.
3. Add tofu and cook until golden brown.
4. Add bell pepper, broccoli, carrot, and zucchini. Stir-fry until vegetables are tender.
5. Drizzle with sesame oil before serving.

Nutrition Information (per serving):

- Calories: 250
- Protein: 15g
- Carbohydrates: 15g
- Fat: 15g
- Fiber: 5g
- Sugar: 5g
- Portion size: 1 cup

Spicy Chickpea Wraps

Ingredients:

- 1 can chickpeas, drained and rinsed
- 1 tbsp olive oil
- 1 tsp chili powder
- 1/2 tsp cumin

- 1/2 tsp paprika

- 1/4 tsp cayenne pepper

- Salt and pepper to taste

- 4 whole wheat tortillas

- 1 cup shredded lettuce

- 1 tomato, diced

- 1/2 red onion, sliced

- 1 avocado, sliced

Instructions:

1. In a pan, heat olive oil and add chickpeas, chili powder, cumin, paprika, cayenne, salt, and pepper.

2. Cook until chickpeas are crispy.

3. In each tortilla, layer chickpeas, lettuce, tomato, red onion, and avocado.

4. Roll up the tortillas to form wraps.

Nutrition Information (per wrap):

- Calories: 320

- Protein: 12g

- Carbohydrates: 45g

- Fat: 10g

- Fiber: 10g

- Sugar: 5g

- Portion size: 1 wrap

Vegan Caesar Salad with Crispy Chickpeas

Ingredients:

- 1 head romaine lettuce, chopped
- 1 can chickpeas, drained and rinsed
- 2 tbsp olive oil
- 1 tsp garlic powder
- 1/2 tsp paprika
- Salt and pepper to taste
- 1/4 cup vegan Caesar dressing
- 2 tbsp nutritional yeast
- 1 lemon, cut into wedges

Instructions:

1. Preheat oven to 400°F. Toss chickpeas with olive oil, garlic powder, paprika, salt, and pepper.
2. Spread chickpeas on a baking sheet and roast for 20 minutes.
3. In a bowl, combine romaine lettuce, vegan Caesar dressing, and nutritional yeast.
4. Top with crispy chickpeas and serve with lemon wedges.

Nutrition Information (per serving):

- Calories: 250
- Protein: 10g
- Carbohydrates: 20g
- Fat: 14g
- Fiber: 8g
- Sugar: 2g
- Portion size: 1 bowl

Lentil and Vegetable Stuffed Peppers

Ingredients:

- 4 bell peppers, tops cut off and seeds removed
- 1 cup cooked lentils
- 1 zucchini, diced
- 1 carrot, diced
- 1 onion, chopped
- 2 cloves garlic, minced
- 1 can diced tomatoes
- 1 tsp Italian seasoning
- Salt and pepper to taste

Instructions:

1. Preheat oven to 375°F.

2. In a pan, sauté onion, garlic, zucchini, and carrot until tender.

3. Add cooked lentils, diced tomatoes, Italian seasoning, salt, and pepper. Simmer for 10 minutes.

4. Stuff bell peppers with lentil mixture and place in a baking dish.

5. Bake for 30 minutes.

Nutrition Information (per pepper):

- Calories: 180
- Protein: 8g
- Carbohydrates: 30g
- Fat: 3g
- Fiber: 10g
- Sugar: 8g
- Portion size: 1 stuffed pepper

Edamame and Quinoa Salad

Ingredients:

- 1 cup cooked quinoa
- 1 cup shelled edamame
- 1 red bell pepper, diced
- 1/2 cucumber, diced
- 2 green onions, sliced

- 2 tbsp rice vinegar

- 1 tbsp soy sauce

- 1 tbsp sesame oil

- 1 tsp maple syrup

Instructions:

1. In a bowl, combine quinoa, edamame, bell pepper, cucumber, and green onions.

2. In a small bowl, whisk together rice vinegar, soy sauce, sesame oil, and maple syrup.

3. Pour the dressing over the salad and toss to combine.

Nutrition Information (per serving):

- Calories: 220

- Protein: 10g

- Carbohydrates: 28g

- Fat: 8g

- Fiber: 5g

- Sugar: 4g

- Portion size: 1 cup

Vegan Sushi Rolls with Brown Rice

Ingredients:

- 2 cups cooked brown rice
- 4 nori sheets
- 1 avocado, sliced
- 1 cucumber, julienned
- 1 carrot, julienned
- 1/4 cup pickled ginger
- Soy sauce for dipping

Instructions:

1. Place a nori sheet on a bamboo sushi mat.
2. Spread a thin layer of brown rice over the nori sheet.
3. Arrange avocado, cucumber, carrot, and pickled ginger in a line along one edge.
4. Roll the sushi tightly using the mat and cut into pieces.
5. Serve with soy sauce.

Nutrition Information (per roll):

- Calories: 180
- Protein: 4g
- Carbohydrates: 30g
- Fat: 6g
- Fiber: 4g

- Sugar: 2g
- Portion size: 1 roll

Chickpea and Spinach Curry

Ingredients:

- 1 can chickpeas, drained and rinsed
- 1 onion, chopped
- 2 cloves garlic, minced
- 1 tbsp ginger, grated
- 1 can coconut milk
- 1 can diced tomatoes
- 2 cups fresh spinach
- 1 tbsp curry powder
- 1 tsp cumin
- Salt and pepper to taste

Instructions:

1. In a pan, sauté onion, garlic, and ginger until fragrant.
2. Add chickpeas, coconut milk, diced tomatoes, curry powder, cumin, salt, and pepper.
3. Simmer for 20 minutes.
4. Stir in spinach and cook until wilted.

Nutrition Information (per serving):

- Calories: 250
- Protein: 8g
- Carbohydrates: 30g
- Fat: 12g
- Fiber: 8g
- Sugar: 6g
- Portion size: 1 cup

Grilled Vegetable and Quinoa Salad

Ingredients:

- 1 cup cooked quinoa
- 1 zucchini, sliced
- 1 bell pepper, sliced
- 1 red onion, sliced
- 1 cup cherry tomatoes
- 2 tbsp olive oil
- 1 tbsp balsamic vinegar
- Salt and pepper to taste

Instructions:

1. Preheat grill to medium-high heat.

2. Toss zucchini, bell pepper, red onion, and cherry tomatoes with olive oil, salt, and pepper.

3. Grill vegetables until tender.

4. In a bowl, combine cooked quinoa, grilled vegetables, and balsamic vinegar.

Nutrition Information (per serving):

- Calories: 210

- Protein: 6g

- Carbohydrates: 32g

- Fat: 8g

- Fiber: 6g

- Sugar: 6g

- Portion size: 1 cup

Spaghetti Squash with Lentil Marinara

Ingredients:

- 1 spaghetti squash

- 1 cup lentils, cooked

- 1 onion, chopped

- 2 cloves garlic, minced

- 1 can crushed tomatoes

- 1 tsp Italian seasoning

- Salt and pepper to taste

Instructions:

1. Preheat oven to 400°F. Cut spaghetti squash in half and remove seeds.
2. Place squash halves cut side down on a baking sheet and bake for 40 minutes.
3. In a pan, sauté onion and garlic until softened. Add lentils, crushed tomatoes, Italian seasoning, salt, and pepper. Simmer for 20 minutes.
4. Scrape the squash into strands and top with lentil marinara.

Nutrition Information (per serving):

- Calories: 200
- Protein: 9g
- Carbohydrates: 40g
- Fat: 2g
- Fiber: 10g
- Sugar: 10g
- Portion size: 1 cup

Zucchini Noodles with Avocado Pesto

Ingredients:

- 2 zucchinis, spiralized
- 1 avocado
- 1 cup fresh basil leaves
- 2 cloves garlic
- 1/4 cup pine nuts
- 2 tbsp olive oil
- Juice of 1 lemon
- Salt and pepper to taste

Instructions:

1. In a food processor, combine avocado, basil, garlic, pine nuts, olive oil, lemon juice, salt, and pepper. Blend until smooth.
2. Toss zucchini noodles with avocado pesto.

Nutrition Information (per serving):

- Calories: 220
- Protein: 4g
- Carbohydrates: 14g
- Fat: 18g
- Fiber: 6g
- Sugar: 4g

- Portion size: 1 cup

Roasted Chickpea and Vegetable Bowl

Ingredients:

- 1 can chickpeas, drained and rinsed
- 1 sweet potato, diced
- 1 bell pepper, chopped
- 1 zucchini, chopped
- 2 tbsp olive oil
- 1 tsp paprika
- 1/2 tsp cumin
- Salt and pepper to taste
- 1 cup cooked quinoa
- 1 avocado, sliced

Instructions:

1. Preheat oven to 400°F. Toss chickpeas, sweet potato, bell pepper, and zucchini with olive oil, paprika, cumin, salt, and pepper.
2. Spread on a baking sheet and roast for 25 minutes.
3. In a bowl, combine roasted vegetables, chickpeas, cooked quinoa, and avocado slices.

Nutrition Information (per bowl):

- Calories: 400
- Protein: 12g
- Carbohydrates: 50g
- Fat: 18g
- Fiber: 10g
- Sugar: 8g
- Portion size: 1 bowl

Chapter 4: Dinner Recipes

Transitioning to a vegan diet while managing type 2 diabetes can seem challenging, but with the right recipes, you can enjoy flavorful, satisfying meals that meet your nutritional needs. Each of these dinner recipes is designed to be high in protein and low in refined carbohydrates, providing essential nutrients while keeping your blood sugar levels stable.

Lentil Shepherd's Pie

Ingredients:

- 1 cup green or brown lentils, rinsed
- 4 cups vegetable broth
- 1 onion, diced
- 2 carrots, diced
- 1 cup peas
- 2 garlic cloves, minced
- 2 tablespoons tomato paste
- 1 teaspoon thyme
- 1 teaspoon rosemary
- 4 cups mashed potatoes (prepared with plant-based milk and vegan butter)

Instructions:

1. Cook lentils in vegetable broth until tender, about 20 minutes.
2. Sauté onion, carrots, and garlic in a large pan until softened.
3. Add lentils, tomato paste, thyme, and rosemary. Stir well.
4. Stir in peas and cook for another 5 minutes.
5. Transfer mixture to a baking dish and top with mashed potatoes.
6. Bake at 375°F for 20 minutes, until the top is golden.

Nutrition Information:

- Calories: 320
- Protein: 12g
- Carbohydrates: 58g
- Fat: 6g
- Fiber: 10g
- Sugar: 5g
- Portion Size: 1 serving

Vegan Stuffed Bell Peppers

Ingredients:

- 4 bell peppers, tops cut off and seeds removed
- 1 cup quinoa, rinsed

- 2 cups vegetable broth
- 1 can black beans, drained and rinsed
- 1 cup corn kernels
- 1 tomato, diced
- 1 teaspoon cumin
- 1 teaspoon paprika
- Salt and pepper to taste

Instructions:

1. Cook quinoa in vegetable broth according to package instructions.
2. Mix cooked quinoa with black beans, corn, tomato, cumin, paprika, salt, and pepper.
3. Stuff the mixture into bell peppers.
4. Place stuffed peppers in a baking dish and cover with foil.
5. Bake at 375°F for 25-30 minutes.

Nutrition Information:

- Calories: 250
- Protein: 10g
- Carbohydrates: 45g
- Fat: 3g
- Fiber: 10g
- Sugar: 8g

- Portion Size: 1 stuffed pepper

Chickpea and Sweet Potato Curry

Ingredients:

- 1 tablespoon olive oil
- 1 onion, diced
- 2 garlic cloves, minced
- 1 tablespoon curry powder
- 1 teaspoon ground turmeric
- 1 can coconut milk
- 2 sweet potatoes, peeled and diced
- 1 can chickpeas, drained and rinsed
- 1 cup spinach leaves

Instructions:

1. Heat olive oil in a large pot over medium heat. Sauté onion and garlic until soft.
2. Stir in curry powder and turmeric and cook for another minute.
3. Add coconut milk and sweet potatoes. Simmer until sweet potatoes are tender.
4. Stir in chickpeas and spinach, cooking until spinach is wilted.

Nutrition Information:

- Calories: 350
- Protein: 9g
- Carbohydrates: 53g
- Fat: 15g
- Fiber: 10g
- Sugar: 10g
- Portion Size: 1 serving

Tofu and Broccoli Stir-Fry

Ingredients:

- 1 block firm tofu, pressed and cubed
- 2 cups broccoli florets
- 1 red bell pepper, sliced
- 3 tablespoons soy sauce
- 1 tablespoon sesame oil
- 1 tablespoon cornstarch
- 1 tablespoon water

Instructions:

1. Heat sesame oil in a large pan over medium-high heat. Add tofu and cook until golden brown.
2. Add broccoli and bell pepper, stir-frying until tender.

3. Mix soy sauce, cornstarch, and water. Pour over vegetables and tofu.

4. Cook until sauce thickens, about 2 minutes.

Nutrition Information:

- Calories: 230
- Protein: 15g
- Carbohydrates: 15g
- Fat: 12g
- Fiber: 4g
- Sugar: 3g
- Portion Size: 1 serving

Vegan Black Bean Burgers

Ingredients:

- 1 can black beans, drained and rinsed
- 1/2 cup breadcrumbs
- 1/4 cup finely chopped onion
- 1 garlic clove, minced
- 1 tablespoon ground flaxseed mixed with 3 tablespoons water
- 1 teaspoon cumin
- Salt and pepper to taste

Instructions:

1. Mash black beans in a bowl until mostly smooth.
2. Mix in breadcrumbs, onion, garlic, flaxseed mixture, cumin, salt, and pepper.
3. Form into patties and cook in a non-stick skillet over medium heat until both sides are browned.

Nutrition Information:

- Calories: 200
- Protein: 8g
- Carbohydrates: 32g
- Fat: 4g
- Fiber: 10g
- Sugar: 1g
- Portion Size: 1 burger

Eggplant and Chickpea Stew

Ingredients:

- 1 tablespoon olive oil
- 1 onion, diced
- 2 garlic cloves, minced
- 1 large eggplant, cubed
- 1 can diced tomatoes

- 1 can chickpeas, drained and rinsed
- 1 teaspoon cumin
- 1 teaspoon paprika
- Salt and pepper to taste

Instructions:

1. Heat olive oil in a large pot over medium heat. Sauté onion and garlic until soft.
2. Add eggplant and cook until browned.
3. Stir in tomatoes, chickpeas, cumin, paprika, salt, and pepper.
4. Simmer for 20 minutes, until eggplant is tender.

Nutrition Information:

- Calories: 250
- Protein: 7g
- Carbohydrates: 32g
- Fat: 10g
- Fiber: 10g
- Sugar: 10g
- Portion Size: 1 serving

Quinoa-Stuffed Acorn Squash

Ingredients:

- 2 acorn squashes, halved and seeded
- 1 cup quinoa, rinsed
- 2 cups vegetable broth
- 1/4 cup dried cranberries
- 1/4 cup chopped pecans
- 1 teaspoon cinnamon
- Salt and pepper to taste

Instructions:

1. Bake acorn squash halves at 400°F for 40 minutes, until tender.
2. Cook quinoa in vegetable broth according to package instructions.
3. Mix quinoa with cranberries, pecans, cinnamon, salt, and pepper.
4. Stuff quinoa mixture into acorn squash halves.

Nutrition Information:

- Calories: 320
- Protein: 7g
- Carbohydrates: 62g
- Fat: 8g

- Fiber: 8g

- Sugar: 12g

- Portion Size: 1 stuffed squash half

Vegan Chili with Lentils and Beans

Ingredients:

- 1 tablespoon olive oil

- 1 onion, diced

- 2 garlic cloves, minced

- 1 bell pepper, diced

- 1 can diced tomatoes

- 1 cup lentils, rinsed

- 1 can black beans, drained and rinsed

- 1 can kidney beans, drained and rinsed

- 2 tablespoons chili powder

- 1 teaspoon cumin

- Salt and pepper to taste

Instructions:

1. Heat olive oil in a large pot over medium heat. Sauté onion, garlic, and bell pepper until soft.

2. Add tomatoes, lentils, beans, chili powder, cumin, salt, and pepper.

3. Simmer for 30 minutes, until lentils are tender.

Nutrition Information:

- Calories: 280
- Protein: 15g
- Carbohydrates: 45g
- Fat: 5g
- Fiber: 15g
- Sugar: 7g
- Portion Size: 1 serving

Grilled Portobello Mushrooms with Quinoa

Ingredients:

- 4 large portobello mushrooms, stems removed
- 1/4 cup balsamic vinegar
- 1 tablespoon olive oil
- 2 garlic cloves, minced
- 1 cup quinoa, rinsed
- 2 cups vegetable broth

Instructions:

1. Marinate mushrooms in balsamic vinegar, olive oil, and garlic for 30 minutes.

2. Cook quinoa in vegetable broth according to package instructions.

3. Grill mushrooms over medium heat for 5-7 minutes on each side.

4. Serve mushrooms over cooked quinoa.

Nutrition Information:

- Calories: 220
- Protein: 7g
- Carbohydrates: 34g
- Fat: 7g
- Fiber: 4g
- Sugar: 4g
- Portion Size: 1 serving

Thai Peanut Tofu and Vegetable Noodles

Ingredients:

- 1 block firm tofu, pressed and cubed
- 2 cups mixed vegetables (carrots, bell peppers, snap peas)
- 1 package rice noodles

- 1/4 cup peanut butter
- 2 tablespoons soy sauce
- 1 tablespoon lime juice
- 1 teaspoon ginger, grated
- 1 garlic clove, minced

Instructions:

1. Cook rice noodles according to package instructions.
2. Sauté tofu and vegetables in a pan until vegetables are tender.
3. Mix peanut butter, soy sauce, lime juice, ginger, and garlic in a bowl.
4. Toss noodles, tofu, and vegetables with peanut sauce.

Nutrition Information:

- Calories: 380
- Protein: 15g
- Carbohydrates: 48g
- Fat: 15g
- Fiber: 6g
- Sugar: 4g
- Portion Size: 1 serving

Spaghetti with Lentil Bolognese

Ingredients:

- 1 cup lentils, rinsed
- 1 can diced tomatoes
- 1 onion, diced
- 2 garlic cloves, minced
- 2 carrots, diced
- 2 celery stalks, diced
- 1 tablespoon olive oil
- 1 teaspoon oregano
- 1 teaspoon basil
- 8 oz whole wheat spaghetti

Instructions:

1. Cook lentils in water until tender, about 20 minutes.
2. Sauté onion, garlic, carrots, and celery in olive oil until soft.
3. Add tomatoes, lentils, oregano, and basil. Simmer for 15 minutes.
4. Cook spaghetti according to package instructions and serve with lentil bolognese.

Nutrition Information:

- Calories: 400
- Protein: 18g

- Carbohydrates: 68g
- Fat: 6g
- Fiber: 14g
- Sugar: 10g
- Portion Size: 1 serving

Baked Tempeh with Vegetables

Ingredients:

- 1 block tempeh, cubed
- 2 cups mixed vegetables (broccoli, carrots, bell peppers)
- 1 tablespoon olive oil
- 2 tablespoons soy sauce
- 1 tablespoon maple syrup
- 1 teaspoon garlic powder

Instructions:

1. Preheat oven to 375°F.
2. Toss tempeh and vegetables with olive oil, soy sauce, maple syrup, and garlic powder.
3. Spread mixture on a baking sheet and bake for 25-30 minutes.

Nutrition Information:

- Calories: 250
- Protein: 14g
- Carbohydrates: 20g
- Fat: 12g
- Fiber: 7g
- Sugar: 6g
- Portion Size: 1 serving

Vegan Paella with Chickpeas and Vegetables

Ingredients:

- 1 tablespoon olive oil
- 1 onion, diced
- 2 garlic cloves, minced
- 1 bell pepper, diced
- 1 cup rice
- 2 cups vegetable broth
- 1 can diced tomatoes
- 1 can chickpeas, drained and rinsed
- 1 teaspoon smoked paprika
- 1 teaspoon turmeric
- Salt and pepper to taste

Instructions:

1. Heat olive oil in a large pan over medium heat. Sauté onion, garlic, and bell pepper until soft.

2. Add rice, vegetable broth, tomatoes, chickpeas, paprika, turmeric, salt, and pepper.

3. Bring to a boil, then reduce heat and simmer until rice is cooked, about 20 minutes.

Nutrition Information:

- Calories: 300
- Protein: 10g
- Carbohydrates: 50g
- Fat: 6g
- Fiber: 8g
- Sugar: 7g
- Portion Size: 1 serving

Stuffed Zucchini Boats with Quinoa

Ingredients:

- 4 zucchini, halved and seeds scooped out
- 1 cup quinoa, rinsed
- 2 cups vegetable broth
- 1 tomato, diced

- 1 can black beans, drained and rinsed
- 1 teaspoon cumin
- 1 teaspoon paprika
- Salt and pepper to taste

Instructions:

1. Cook quinoa in vegetable broth according to package instructions.
2. Mix quinoa with tomato, black beans, cumin, paprika, salt, and pepper.
3. Stuff the mixture into zucchini halves.
4. Place stuffed zucchini in a baking dish and bake at 375°F for 20-25 minutes.

Nutrition Information:

- Calories: 220
- Protein: 8g
- Carbohydrates: 36g
- Fat: 4g
- Fiber: 8g
- Sugar: 6g
- Portion Size: 1 stuffed zucchini half

Cauliflower and Chickpea Tacos

Ingredients:

- 1 head cauliflower, chopped into florets
- 1 can chickpeas, drained and rinsed
- 2 tablespoons olive oil
- 1 teaspoon cumin
- 1 teaspoon paprika
- 1 teaspoon garlic powder
- Salt and pepper to taste
- 8 small corn tortillas
- Optional toppings: avocado, salsa, cilantro

Instructions:

1. Preheat oven to 400°F.
2. Toss cauliflower and chickpeas with olive oil, cumin, paprika, garlic powder, salt, and pepper.
3. Spread mixture on a baking sheet and roast for 25-30 minutes.
4. Serve roasted cauliflower and chickpeas in tortillas with desired toppings.

Nutrition Information:

- Calories: 250
- Protein: 8g

- Carbohydrates: 38g

- Fat: 8g

- Fiber: 8g

- Sugar: 4g

- Portion Size: 2 tacos

Chapter 5: Snacks and Appetizers

Finding nutritious, delicious snacks and appetizers can be a challenge, especially for those managing Type 2 diabetes. This chapter offers a variety of high-protein, vegan options that are not only healthy but also satisfying and flavorful.

Roasted Chickpeas

Ingredients:

- 1 can chickpeas, drained and rinsed
- 1 tbsp olive oil
- 1 tsp paprika
- 1 tsp garlic powder
- 1/2 tsp salt

Instructions:

1. Preheat oven to 400°F (200°C).
2. Toss chickpeas with olive oil, paprika, garlic powder, and salt.
3. Spread on a baking sheet and roast for 25-30 minutes, shaking halfway through.

Nutrition Information (per serving):

- Calories: 180
- Protein: 8g
- Carbohydrates: 30g
- Fat: 6g
- Fiber: 8g
- Sugar: 2g
- Portion Size: 1/2 cup

Veggie Sticks with Hummus

Ingredients:

- 1 cup baby carrots
- 1 cup cucumber sticks
- 1 cup bell pepper strips
- 1 cup cherry tomatoes
- 1 cup hummus

Instructions:

1. Arrange the vegetable sticks and cherry tomatoes on a platter.
2. Serve with a bowl of hummus.

Nutrition Information (per serving):

- Calories: 150
- Protein: 5g
- Carbohydrates: 20g
- Fat: 7g
- Fiber: 6g
- Sugar: 5g
- Portion Size: 1 cup veggies + 1/4 cup hummus

Spicy Edamame

Ingredients:

- 2 cups edamame, in pods
- 1 tbsp soy sauce
- 1 tsp sriracha
- 1 tsp sesame oil

Instructions:

1. Steam edamame until tender, about 5 minutes.
2. Toss with soy sauce, sriracha, and sesame oil.

Nutrition Information (per serving):

- Calories: 120
- Protein: 11g

- Carbohydrates: 10g

- Fat: 5g

- Fiber: 4g

- Sugar: 1g

- Portion Size: 1 cup

Vegan Stuffed Mushrooms

Ingredients:

- 12 large mushrooms, stems removed

- 1/2 cup cooked quinoa

- 1/4 cup nutritional yeast

- 1 tbsp olive oil

- 1 clove garlic, minced

- Salt and pepper to taste

Instructions:

1. Preheat oven to 375°F (190°C).

2. Mix quinoa, nutritional yeast, olive oil, garlic, salt, and pepper.

3. Stuff each mushroom with the quinoa mixture.

4. Bake for 20 minutes.

Nutrition Information (per serving):

- Calories: 90

- Protein: 4g

- Carbohydrates: 8g

- Fat: 4g

- Fiber: 2g

- Sugar: 2g

- Portion Size: 3 mushrooms

Almond Flour Crackers with Guacamole

Ingredients:

- 1 cup almond flour

- 1 tbsp flaxseed meal

- 1/2 tsp salt

- 2 tbsp water

- 1 ripe avocado

- 1 tbsp lime juice

- 1/4 cup diced tomato

- Salt and pepper to taste

Instructions:

1. Preheat oven to 350°F (175°C).

2. Mix almond flour, flaxseed meal, salt, and water to form a dough.

3. Roll out the dough thinly and cut into crackers.

4. Bake for 15 minutes.

5. Mash avocado with lime juice, tomato, salt, and pepper for guacamole.

Nutrition Information (per serving):

- Calories: 200
- Protein: 6g
- Carbohydrates: 10g
- Fat: 16g
- Fiber: 6g
- Sugar: 1g
- Portion Size: 10 crackers + 1/4 cup guacamole

Baked Tofu Bites

Ingredients:

- 1 block firm tofu, drained and cubed
- 2 tbsp soy sauce
- 1 tbsp olive oil
- 1 tsp garlic powder
- 1 tsp smoked paprika

Instructions:

1. Preheat oven to 400°F (200°C).

2. Toss tofu cubes with soy sauce, olive oil, garlic powder, and smoked paprika.

3. Spread on a baking sheet and bake for 25 minutes, turning halfway.

Nutrition Information (per serving):

- Calories: 160
- Protein: 12g
- Carbohydrates: 6g
- Fat: 10g
- Fiber: 2g
- Sugar: 1g
- Portion Size: 1/2 cup

Kale Chips

Ingredients:

- 1 bunch kale, stems removed and torn into pieces
- 1 tbsp olive oil
- 1/2 tsp salt

Instructions:

1. Preheat oven to 350°F (175°C).

2. Toss kale with olive oil and salt.

3. Spread on a baking sheet and bake for 15 minutes, until crisp.

Nutrition Information (per serving):

- Calories: 50
- Protein: 3g
- Carbohydrates: 7g
- Fat: 2g
- Fiber: 2g
- Sugar: 0g
- Portion Size: 1 cup

Lentil and Veggie Spring Rolls

Ingredients:

- 8 rice paper wraps
- 1 cup cooked lentils
- 1 cup shredded carrots
- 1 cup thinly sliced bell peppers
- 1 cup fresh spinach
- 1/4 cup chopped fresh herbs (mint, cilantro)

Instructions:

1. Soak rice paper wraps in warm water until soft.
2. Fill each wrap with lentils, carrots, bell peppers, spinach, and herbs.
3. Roll tightly and serve.

Nutrition Information (per serving):

- Calories: 120
- Protein: 6g
- Carbohydrates: 20g
- Fat: 1g
- Fiber: 4g
- Sugar: 2g
- Portion Size: 2 rolls

Vegan Cheese Dip with Crudités

Ingredients:

- 1 cup cashews, soaked
- 1/4 cup nutritional yeast
- 1/2 cup water
- 1 clove garlic
- 1 tbsp lemon juice
- Assorted raw vegetables (carrots, celery, bell peppers)

Instructions:

1. Blend cashews, nutritional yeast, water, garlic, and lemon juice until smooth.

2. Serve with assorted raw vegetables.

Nutrition Information (per serving):

- Calories: 180

- Protein: 6g

- Carbohydrates: 12g

- Fat: 12g

- Fiber: 3g

- Sugar: 3g

- Portion Size: 1/4 cup dip – 1 cup veggies

Stuffed Mini Peppers with Hummus

Ingredients:

- 12 mini bell peppers, halved and seeded

- 1 cup hummus

Instructions:

1. Fill each mini pepper half with hummus.

2. Arrange on a platter and serve.

Nutrition Information (per serving):

- Calories: 80
- Protein: 3g
- Carbohydrates: 10g
- Fat: 4g
- Fiber: 3g
- Sugar: 3g
- Portion Size: 4 halves

Zucchini Fritters

Ingredients:

- 2 zucchinis, grated
- 1/4 cup chickpea flour
- 1/4 cup nutritional yeast
- 1 clove garlic, minced
- Salt and pepper to taste
- 2 tbsp olive oil

Instructions:

1. Mix grated zucchini, chickpea flour, nutritional yeast, garlic, salt, and pepper.
2. Form into small patties.

3. Heat olive oil in a pan and cook patties until golden brown, about 4 minutes per side.

Nutrition Information (per serving):

- Calories: 120
- Protein: 5g
- Carbohydrates: 10g
- Fat: 7g
- Fiber: 2g
- Sugar: 2g
- Portion Size: 3 fritters

Spicy Roasted Cauliflower

Ingredients:

- 1 head cauliflower, cut into florets
- 2 tbsp olive oil
- 1 tsp chili powder
- 1/2 tsp cumin
- Salt to taste

Instructions:

1. Preheat oven to 400°F (200°C).

2. Toss cauliflower with olive oil, chili powder, cumin, and salt.

3. Spread on a baking sheet and roast for 25 minutes, until tender.

Nutrition Information (per serving):

- Calories: 100
- Protein: 3g
- Carbohydrates: 10g
- Fat: 7g
- Fiber: 4g
- Sugar: 2g
- Portion Size: 1 cup

Vegan Spinach Artichoke Dip

Ingredients:

- 1 cup raw cashews, soaked
- 1 cup fresh spinach, chopped
- 1/2 cup artichoke hearts, chopped
- 1 clove garlic
- 1 tbsp lemon juice
- 1/4 cup nutritional yeast
- Salt and pepper to taste

Instructions:

1. Blend cashews, garlic, lemon juice, and nutritional yeast until smooth.
2. Stir in chopped spinach and artichoke hearts.
3. Season with salt and pepper.

Nutrition Information (per serving):

- Calories: 150
- Protein: 5g
- Carbohydrates: 10g
- Fat: 10g
- Fiber: 3g
- Sugar: 1g
- Portion Size: 1/4 cup

Avocado and Black Bean Salsa

Ingredients:

- 1 avocado, diced
- 1 cup black beans, rinsed and drained
- 1/2 cup diced tomatoes
- 1/4 cup chopped red onion
- 1 tbsp lime juice
- Salt and pepper to taste

Instructions:

1. Mix avocado, black beans, tomatoes, red onion, and lime juice.

2. Season with salt and pepper.

Nutrition Information (per serving):

- Calories: 160
- Protein: 5g
- Carbohydrates: 18g
- Fat: 8g
- Fiber: 8g
- Sugar: 2g
- Portion Size: 1/2 cup

Sweet Potato Bites with Avocado

Ingredients:

- 1 large sweet potato, sliced into rounds
- 1 tbsp olive oil
- 1 ripe avocado
- 1 tbsp lime juice
- Salt and pepper to taste

Instructions:

1. Preheat oven to 400°F (200°C).
2. Toss sweet potato rounds with olive oil and roast for 20 minutes.
3. Mash avocado with lime juice, salt, and pepper.
4. Top each sweet potato round with mashed avocado.

Nutrition Information (per serving):

- Calories: 180
- Protein: 3g
- Carbohydrates: 25g
- Fat: 8g
- Fiber: 6g
- Sugar: 5g
- Portion Size: 5 rounds

Chapter 6: Desserts

In this chapter, we present delectable dessert recipes that are both high in protein and suitable for individuals with type 2 diabetes. From creamy puddings to fruity sorbets and decadent cakes, these recipes offer a variety of sweet treats to satisfy your cravings while still supporting your health goals.

Chia Seed Pudding with Coconut Milk

Ingredients:

- 1/4 cup chia seeds
- 1 cup unsweetened coconut milk
- 1 tablespoon maple syrup (optional)
- Fresh berries for topping

Instructions:

1. In a bowl, mix chia seeds and coconut milk together. Stir well to combine.
2. Add maple syrup if desired for sweetness.
3. Cover and refrigerate for at least 4 hours or overnight, until pudding is thickened.
4. Serve topped with fresh berries.

Nutrition Information (per serving):

- Calories: 180
- Protein: 4g
- Carbohydrates: 15g
- Fat: 12g
- Fiber: 10g
- Sugar: 3g
- Portion Size: 1/2 cup

Vegan Protein Brownies

Ingredients:

- 1 cup cooked black beans
- 1/2 cup almond butter
- 1/4 cup maple syrup
- 1/4 cup cocoa powder
- 1 scoop vegan protein powder
- 1 teaspoon vanilla extract

Instructions:

1. Preheat oven to 350°F (175°C). Grease a baking dish.
2. In a food processor, blend black beans, almond butter, maple syrup, cocoa powder, protein powder, and vanilla extract until smooth.

3. Spread mixture evenly into the prepared baking dish.

4. Bake for 20-25 minutes, or until edges are firm.

5. Allow to cool before cutting into squares.

Nutrition Information (per serving):

- Calories: 120
- Protein: 6g
- Carbohydrates: 15g
- Fat: 5g
- Fiber: 5g
- Sugar: 5g
- Portion Size: 1 brownie

Almond Butter and Dark Chocolate Energy Balls

Ingredients:

- 1 cup rolled oats
- 1/2 cup almond butter
- 1/4 cup dark chocolate chips
- 1/4 cup maple syrup
- 1 teaspoon vanilla extract
- Pinch of sea salt

Instructions:

1. In a large mixing bowl, combine rolled oats, almond butter, dark chocolate chips, maple syrup, vanilla extract, and a pinch of sea salt.
2. Mix until well combined and the mixture sticks together.
3. Roll the mixture into small balls using your hands.
4. Place the energy balls on a baking sheet lined with parchment paper.
5. Refrigerate for at least 30 minutes before serving.

Nutrition Information (per serving, 2 energy balls):

- Calories: 180
- Protein: 5g
- Carbohydrates: 20g
- Fat: 10g
- Fiber: 3g
- Sugar: 8g
- Portion Size: 2 energy balls

Baked Apple Slices with Cinnamon

Ingredients:

- 2 apples, sliced
- 1 teaspoon cinnamon

- 1 tablespoon maple syrup (optional)

Instructions:

1. Preheat oven to 375°F (190°C).

2. Place apple slices in a baking dish.

3. Sprinkle cinnamon over the apple slices. Drizzle with maple syrup if desired.

4. Bake for 20-25 minutes, or until apples are tender.

5. Serve warm as is or with a dollop of vegan yogurt.

Nutrition Information (per serving):

- Calories: 70
- Protein: 0g
- Carbohydrates: 20g
- Fat: 0g
- Fiber: 4g
- Sugar: 15g
- Portion Size: 1/2 cup

Vegan Chocolate Avocado Mousse

Ingredients:

- 2 ripe avocados
- 1/4 cup cocoa powder

- 1/4 cup maple syrup

- 1 teaspoon vanilla extract

- Pinch of sea salt

Instructions:

1. In a food processor, blend avocados, cocoa powder, maple syrup, vanilla extract, and a pinch of sea salt until smooth and creamy.

2. Transfer the mousse to serving dishes.

3. Refrigerate for at least 30 minutes before serving.

Nutrition Information (per serving):

- Calories: 150

- Protein: 2g

- Carbohydrates: 15g

- Fat: 10g

- Fiber: 6g

- Sugar: 6g

- Portion Size: 1/2 cup

Coconut and Almond Flour Cookies

Ingredients:

- 1 cup almond flour

- 1/4 cup coconut flour
- 1/4 cup coconut oil, melted
- 1/4 cup maple syrup
- 1 teaspoon vanilla extract
- Pinch of sea salt
- Unsweetened shredded coconut for topping (optional)

Instructions:

1. Preheat oven to 350°F (175°C). Line a baking sheet with parchment paper.
2. In a mixing bowl, combine almond flour, coconut flour, melted coconut oil, maple syrup, vanilla extract, and a pinch of sea salt.
3. Mix until a dough forms.
4. Roll the dough into balls and flatten them on the prepared baking sheet.
5. Sprinkle shredded coconut on top if desired.
6. Bake for 12-15 minutes, or until edges are golden brown.
7. Allow to cool before serving.

Nutrition Information (per serving, 2 cookies):

- Calories: 160
- Protein: 3g
- Carbohydrates: 10g

- Fat: 12g
- Fiber: 2g
- Sugar: 6g
- Portion Size: 2 cookies

Berry Crumble with Oat Topping

Ingredients:

- 2 cups mixed berries (such as strawberries, blueberries, and raspberries)
- 1 tablespoon maple syrup
- 1/2 cup rolled oats
- 1/4 cup almond flour
- 2 tablespoons coconut oil, melted
- 1 tablespoon maple syrup
- 1/2 teaspoon cinnamon
- Pinch of sea salt

Instructions:

1. Preheat oven to 350°F (175°C). Grease a baking dish.
2. In a bowl, toss mixed berries with 1 tablespoon of maple syrup. Spread evenly in the prepared baking dish.

3. In another bowl, combine rolled oats, almond flour, melted coconut oil, 1 tablespoon of maple syrup, cinnamon, and a pinch of sea salt. Mix until crumbly.

4. Sprinkle the oat mixture over the berries.

5. Bake for 25-30 minutes, or until the topping is golden brown and the berries are bubbling.

6. Serve warm, optionally with a scoop of vegan ice cream.

Nutrition Information (per serving):

- Calories: 180
- Protein: 3g
- Carbohydrates: 25g
- Fat: 8g
- Fiber: 5g
- Sugar: 12g
- Portion Size: 1/2 cup

Vegan Banana Bread

Ingredients:

- 2 ripe bananas, mashed
- 1/4 cup coconut oil, melted
- 1/4 cup maple syrup
- 1 teaspoon vanilla extract

- 1 1/2 cups whole wheat flour
- 1 teaspoon baking powder
- 1/2 teaspoon baking soda
- 1/2 teaspoon cinnamon
- Pinch of sea salt
- Optional: chopped nuts or chocolate chips for topping

Instructions:

1. Preheat oven to 350°F (175°C). Grease a loaf pan.
2. In a large mixing bowl, combine mashed bananas, melted coconut oil, maple syrup, and vanilla extract.
3. In a separate bowl, whisk together whole wheat flour, baking powder, baking soda, cinnamon, and a pinch of sea salt.
4. Gradually add the dry ingredients to the wet ingredients, stirring until just combined.
5. Pour the batter into the prepared loaf pan.
6. If desired, sprinkle chopped nuts or chocolate chips on top.
7. Bake for 45-50 minutes, or until a toothpick inserted into the center comes out clean.
8. Allow to cool before slicing.

Nutrition Information (per serving, 1 slice):
- Calories: 160
- Protein: 3g

- Carbohydrates: 20g

- Fat: 7g

- Fiber: 3g

- Sugar: 7g

- Portion Size: 1 slice

Chocolate Chia Seed Pudding

Ingredients:

- 1/4 cup chia seeds

- 1 cup unsweetened almond milk

- 2 tablespoons cocoa powder

- 1-2 tablespoons maple syrup (adjust to taste)

- Optional toppings: sliced bananas, chopped nuts, shredded coconut

Instructions:

1. In a bowl, whisk together chia seeds, almond milk, cocoa powder, and maple syrup until well combined.

2. Let the mixture sit for 5 minutes, then whisk again to prevent clumping.

3. Cover and refrigerate for at least 2 hours, or preferably overnight, until pudding is thickened.

4. Serve chilled with your favorite toppings.

Nutrition Information (per serving):

- Calories: 120
- Protein: 4g
- Carbohydrates: 15g
- Fat: 6g
- Fiber: 7g
- Sugar: 5g
- Portion Size: 1/2 cup

Raw Vegan Cheesecake

Ingredients: For the crust:

- 1 cup almonds
- 1 cup dates, pitted
- Pinch of sea salt

For the filling:

- 2 cups cashews, soaked for 4-6 hours
- 1/2 cup coconut cream
- 1/4 cup lemon juice
- 1/4 cup maple syrup
- 1 teaspoon vanilla extract
- Pinch of sea salt

Instructions:

1. In a food processor, blend almonds, dates, and a pinch of sea salt until mixture sticks together.

2. Press the mixture into the bottom of a greased springform pan to form the crust. Place in the freezer while preparing the filling.

3. Rinse soaked cashews and drain well. In a blender, combine cashews, coconut cream, lemon juice, maple syrup, vanilla extract, and a pinch of sea salt. Blend until smooth and creamy.

4. Pour the filling over the crust in the springform pan.

5. Smooth the top with a spatula.

6. Place the cheesecake in the freezer for at least 4 hours, or until set.

7. Before serving, let the cheesecake thaw for 10-15 minutes. Slice and enjoy!

Nutrition Information (per serving):

- Calories: 250
- Protein: 6g
- Carbohydrates: 20g
- Fat: 18g
- Fiber: 3g
- Sugar: 12g

- Portion Size: 1 slice

Mango Sorbet

Ingredients:

- 2 cups frozen mango chunks
- 1/4 cup coconut milk
- 1 tablespoon lime juice
- 1 tablespoon maple syrup (optional)

Instructions:

1. In a blender, combine frozen mango chunks, coconut milk, lime juice, and maple syrup.
2. Blend until smooth and creamy, adding more coconut milk if needed to reach desired consistency.
3. Transfer the mixture to a shallow dish and freeze for 2-3 hours, or until firm.
4. Serve scoops of mango sorbet in bowls or cones.

Nutrition Information (per serving):

- Calories: 120
- Protein: 1g
- Carbohydrates: 30g
- Fat: 2g

- Fiber: 3g
- Sugar: 25g
- Portion Size: 1/2 cup

Vegan Carrot Cake

Ingredients: For the cake:

- 2 cups grated carrots
- 1 cup whole wheat flour
- 1/2 cup almond flour
- 1/2 cup chopped walnuts
- 1/2 cup raisins
- 1 teaspoon baking powder
- 1/2 teaspoon baking soda
- 1 teaspoon cinnamon
- 1/4 teaspoon nutmeg
- Pinch of sea salt
- 1/2 cup maple syrup
- 1/4 cup coconut oil, melted
- 1/4 cup unsweetened applesauce
- 1 teaspoon vanilla extract

For the frosting:

- 1 cup raw cashews, soaked for 4-6 hours

- 1/4 cup coconut cream
- 2 tablespoons maple syrup
- 1 tablespoon lemon juice
- 1 teaspoon vanilla extract
- Pinch of sea salt

Instructions:

1. Preheat oven to 350°F (175°C). Grease a cake pan.
2. In a large mixing bowl, combine grated carrots, whole wheat flour, almond flour, chopped walnuts, raisins, baking powder, baking soda, cinnamon, nutmeg, and a pinch of sea salt.
3. In a separate bowl, whisk together maple syrup, melted coconut oil, applesauce, and vanilla extract.
4. Gradually add the wet ingredients to the dry ingredients, stirring until well combined.
5. Pour the batter into the prepared cake pan.
6. Bake for 30-35 minutes, or until a toothpick inserted into the center comes out clean.
7. Let the cake cool completely before frosting.

For the frosting:

1. Rinse soaked cashews and drain well.

2. In a blender, combine soaked cashews, coconut cream, maple syrup, lemon juice, vanilla extract, and a pinch of sea salt.

3. Blend until smooth and creamy.

4. Once the cake has cooled, spread the frosting evenly over the top.

5. Slice and serve.

Nutrition Information (per serving, 1 slice with frosting):

- Calories: 280
- Protein: 6g
- Carbohydrates: 30g
- Fat: 16g
- Fiber: 4g
- Sugar: 16g
- Portion Size: 1 slice

Peanut Butter and Chocolate Smoothie Bowl

Ingredients:

- 1 ripe banana
- 1/4 cup creamy peanut butter
- 1 tablespoon cocoa powder

- 1/2 cup unsweetened almond milk
- 1 tablespoon maple syrup (optional)
- Toppings: sliced banana, chopped peanuts, dark chocolate chips

Instructions:

1. In a blender, combine ripe banana, creamy peanut butter, cocoa powder, unsweetened almond milk, and maple syrup.
2. Blend until smooth and creamy, adding more almond milk if needed to reach desired consistency.
3. Pour the smoothie into a bowl.
4. Top with sliced banana, chopped peanuts, and dark chocolate chips.
5. Enjoy with a spoon!

Nutrition Information (per serving):

- Calories: 350
- Protein: 8g
- Carbohydrates: 25g
- Fat: 22g
- Fiber: 6g
- Sugar: 12g
- Portion Size: 1 smoothie bowl

Vegan Lemon Bars

Ingredients: For the crust:

- 1 cup almond flour
- 1/4 cup coconut oil, melted
- 2 tablespoons maple syrup
- Pinch of sea salt

For the filling:

- 1 cup raw cashews, soaked for 4-6 hours
- 1/2 cup coconut cream
- 1/4 cup lemon juice
- Zest of 1 lemon
- 1/4 cup maple syrup
- 2 tablespoons arrowroot powder

Instructions:

1. Preheat oven to 350°F (175°C). Grease a baking dish.
2. In a mixing bowl, combine almond flour, melted coconut oil, maple syrup, and a pinch of sea salt for the crust. Press the mixture into the bottom of the prepared baking dish.
3. Bake the crust for 10-12 minutes, or until lightly golden brown.

4. In a blender, combine soaked cashews, coconut cream, lemon juice, lemon zest, maple syrup, and arrowroot powder for the filling. Blend until smooth and creamy.

5. Pour the filling over the baked crust.

6. Return the baking dish to the oven and bake for another 20-25 minutes, or until the filling is set.

7. Let the lemon bars cool completely before slicing into squares.

8. Store in the refrigerator until ready to serve.

Nutrition Information (per serving, 1 square):

- Calories: 180
- Protein: 4g
- Carbohydrates: 15g
- Fat: 12g
- Fiber: 2g
- Sugar: 8g
- Portion Size: 1 square

Cinnamon Roasted Chickpeas

Ingredients:

- 1 can (15 ounces) chickpeas, drained and rinsed
- 1 tablespoon coconut oil, melted

- 1 tablespoon maple syrup
- 1 teaspoon ground cinnamon
- Pinch of sea salt

Instructions:

1. Preheat oven to 400°F (200°C). Line a baking sheet with parchment paper.
2. Pat dry the chickpeas with a clean kitchen towel to remove excess moisture.
3. In a bowl, toss the chickpeas with melted coconut oil, maple syrup, ground cinnamon, and a pinch of sea salt until evenly coated.
4. Spread the chickpeas in a single layer on the prepared baking sheet.
5. Roast in the preheated oven for 25-30 minutes, shaking the pan halfway through, until chickpeas are crispy and golden brown.
6. Let the roasted chickpeas cool completely before serving as a crunchy snack.

Nutrition Information (per serving):
- Calories: 120
- Protein: 4g
- Carbohydrates: 15g

- Fat: 5g
- Fiber: 4g
- Sugar: 3g
- Portion Size: 1/4 cup

Chapter 7: Smoothies

In this chapter, we've curated protein-packed smoothie recipes that are not only delicious but also provide a boost of energy and essential nutrients. Whether you're looking for a refreshing morning pick-me-up or a post-workout refuel, these smoothies have got you covered.

Green Protein Smoothie

Ingredients:

- 1 cup spinach
- 1/2 ripe avocado
- 1 scoop plant-based protein powder
- 1/2 frozen banana
- 1 cup almond milk
- Ice cubes (optional)

Instructions:

1. Add all ingredients to a blender.
2. Blend until smooth and creamy.
3. Serve immediately and enjoy!

Nutrition Information (per serving):

- Calories: 250
- Protein: 20g
- Carbohydrates: 20g
- Fat: 10g
- Fiber: 8g
- Sugar: 6g
- Portion size: 1 serving

Berry Protein Smoothie

Ingredients:

- 1/2 cup mixed berries (strawberries, blueberries, raspberries)
- 1/2 cup plain Greek yogurt
- 1 scoop vanilla protein powder
- 1 tablespoon honey or maple syrup (optional)
- 1/2 cup almond milk
- Ice cubes (optional)

Instructions:

1. Combine all ingredients in a blender.
2. Blend until smooth and creamy.
3. Pour into a glass and enjoy!

Nutrition Information (per serving):

- Calories: 220
- Protein: 25g
- Carbohydrates: 25g
- Fat: 3g
- Fiber: 5g
- Sugar: 15g
- Portion size: 1 serving

Peanut Butter Banana Smoothie

Ingredients:

- 1 ripe banana
- 2 tablespoons natural peanut butter
- 1 scoop chocolate protein powder
- 1 cup unsweetened almond milk
- Ice cubes (optional)

Instructions:

1. Peel the banana and place it in a blender.
2. Add peanut butter, protein powder, and almond milk.
3. Blend until smooth and creamy.
4. Serve immediately and enjoy!

Nutrition Information (per serving):

- Calories: 320
- Protein: 25g
- Carbohydrates: 30g
- Fat: 12g
- Fiber: 6g
- Sugar: 12g
- Portion size: 1 serving

Chocolate Protein Smoothie

Ingredients:

- 1 cup unsweetened almond milk
- 1 scoop chocolate protein powder
- 1 tablespoon unsweetened cocoa powder
- 1/2 frozen banana
- 1 tablespoon almond butter
- Ice cubes (optional)

Instructions:

1. Combine all ingredients in a blender.
2. Blend until smooth and creamy.
3. Pour into a glass and enjoy!

Nutrition Information (per serving):

- Calories: 280
- Protein: 30g
- Carbohydrates: 20g
- Fat: 10g
- Fiber: 5g
- Sugar: 8g
- Portion size: 1 serving

Tropical Protein Smoothie

Ingredients:

- 1/2 cup frozen pineapple chunks
- 1/2 cup frozen mango chunks
- 1 scoop vanilla protein powder
- 1/2 cup coconut milk
- 1/2 cup water
- Ice cubes (optional)

Instructions:

1. Place all ingredients in a blender.
2. Blend until smooth and creamy.
3. Pour into a glass and enjoy!

Nutrition Information (per serving):

- Calories: 260
- Protein: 20g
- Carbohydrates: 30g
- Fat: 8g
- Fiber: 5g
- Sugar: 20g
- Portion size: 1 serving

Almond Joy Smoothie

Ingredients:

- 1/2 cup unsweetened almond milk
- 1/2 cup coconut milk
- 1 scoop chocolate protein powder
- 2 tablespoons shredded coconut
- 1 tablespoon almond butter
- Ice cubes (optional)

Instructions:

1. Combine all ingredients in a blender.
2. Blend until smooth and creamy.
3. Pour into a glass and enjoy!

Nutrition Information (per serving):

- Calories: 300
- Protein: 25g
- Carbohydrates: 15g
- Fat: 15g
- Fiber: 5g
- Sugar: 5g
- Portion size: 1 serving

Spinach and Pineapple Smoothie

Ingredients:

- 1 cup fresh spinach
- 1/2 cup frozen pineapple chunks
- 1/2 frozen banana
- 1 scoop vanilla protein powder
- 1/2 cup unsweetened almond milk
- Ice cubes (optional)

Instructions:

1. Add spinach, pineapple, banana, protein powder, and almond milk to a blender.
2. Blend until smooth and creamy.
3. Pour into a glass and enjoy!

Nutrition Information (per serving):

- Calories: 220
- Protein: 20g
- Carbohydrates: 25g
- Fat: 3g
- Fiber: 5g
- Sugar: 15g
- Portion size: 1 serving

Blueberry Almond Smoothie

Ingredients:

- 1/2 cup frozen blueberries
- 1/4 cup almonds
- 1 scoop vanilla protein powder
- 1/2 cup plain Greek yogurt
- 1/2 cup almond milk
- Ice cubes (optional)

Instructions:

1. Combine all ingredients in a blender.
2. Blend until smooth and creamy.
3. Pour into a glass and enjoy!

Nutrition Information (per serving):

- Calories: 280
- Protein: 25g
- Carbohydrates: 20g
- Fat: 12g
- Fiber: 5g
- Sugar: 10g
- Portion size: 1 serving

Vegan Matcha Protein Smoothie

Ingredients:

- 1 teaspoon matcha powder
- 1 scoop vanilla protein powder
- 1/2 cup unsweetened almond milk
- 1/2 frozen banana
- 1 tablespoon maple syrup
- Ice cubes (optional)

Instructions:

1. Place all ingredients in a blender.
2. Blend until smooth and creamy.
3. Pour into a glass and enjoy!

Nutrition Information (per serving):

- Calories: 230
- Protein: 20g
- Carbohydrates: 25g
- Fat: 5g
- Fiber: 4g
- Sugar: 15g
- Portion size: 1 serving

Raspberry and Oat Smoothie

Ingredients:

- 1/2 cup frozen raspberries
- 1/4 cup rolled oats
- 1 scoop vanilla protein powder
- 1/2 cup plain Greek yogurt
- 1/2 cup almond milk
- Ice cubes (optional)

Instructions:

1. Combine all ingredients in a blender.
2. Blend until smooth and creamy.
3. Pour into a glass and enjoy!

Nutrition Information (per serving):

- Calories: 270
- Protein: 25g
- Carbohydrates: 30g
- Fat: 6g
- Fiber: 7g
- Sugar: 10g
- Portion size: 1 serving

Orange and Ginger Smoothie

Ingredients:

- 1 orange, peeled and segmented
- 1 teaspoon grated ginger
- 1 scoop vanilla protein powder
- 1/2 cup plain Greek yogurt
- 1/2 cup almond milk
- Ice cubes (optional)

Instructions:

1. Place all ingredients in a blender.
2. Blend until smooth and creamy.
3. Pour into a glass and enjoy!

Nutrition Information (per serving):

- Calories: 230
- Protein: 20g
- Carbohydrates: 25g
- Fat: 4g
- Fiber: 5g
- Sugar: 15g
- Portion size: 1 serving

Pumpkin Spice Smoothie

Ingredients:

- 1/2 cup pumpkin puree
- 1 scoop vanilla protein powder
- 1/2 teaspoon pumpkin pie spice
- 1 tablespoon maple syrup
- 1/2 cup almond milk
- Ice cubes (optional)

Instructions:

1. Combine all ingredients in a blender.
2. Blend until smooth and creamy.
3. Pour into a glass and enjoy!

Nutrition Information (per serving):

- Calories: 240
- Protein: 20g
- Carbohydrates: 25g
- Fat: 4g
- Fiber: 6g
- Sugar: 10g
- Portion size: 1 serving

Apple Pie Smoothie

Ingredients:

- 1 apple, cored and chopped
- 1 scoop vanilla protein powder
- 1/4 teaspoon ground cinnamon
- 1 tablespoon almond butter
- 1/2 cup unsweetened almond milk
- Ice cubes (optional)

Instructions:

1. Add all ingredients to a blender.
2. Blend until smooth and creamy.
3. Serve immediately and enjoy!

Nutrition Information (per serving):

- Calories: 260
- Protein: 20g
- Carbohydrates: 30g
- Fat: 8g
- Fiber: 6g
- Sugar: 18g
- Portion size: 1 serving

Kiwi and Kale Smoothie

Ingredients:

- 2 kiwis, peeled and chopped
- 1 cup chopped kale leaves
- 1 scoop vanilla protein powder
- 1/2 cup unsweetened almond milk
- 1 tablespoon honey or maple syrup (optional)
- Ice cubes (optional)

Instructions:

1. Place all ingredients in a blender.
2. Blend until smooth and creamy.
3. Pour into a glass and enjoy!

Nutrition Information (per serving):

- Calories: 230
- Protein: 20g
- Carbohydrates: 25g
- Fat: 3g
- Fiber: 7g
- Sugar: 15g
- Portion size: 1 serving

Mango and Turmeric Smoothie

Ingredients:

- 1 cup frozen mango chunks
- 1/2 teaspoon ground turmeric
- 1 scoop vanilla protein powder
- 1/2 cup coconut water
- 1/2 cup unsweetened almond milk
- Ice cubes (optional)

Instructions:

1. Add all ingredients to a blender.
2. Blend until smooth and creamy.
3. Pour into a glass and enjoy!

Nutrition Information (per serving):

- Calories: 250
- Protein: 20g
- Carbohydrates: 30g
- Fat: 3g
- Fiber: 5g
- Sugar: 20g
- Portion size: 1 serving

CONCLUSION

As we conclude this journey through the world of high-protein vegan meals tailored for individuals managing type 2 diabetes, it's essential to reflect on the significance of the knowledge gained and the delicious recipes shared within these pages. Through understanding the interplay between nutrition and health, we've empowered ourselves with the tools to make informed dietary choices that promote well-being and vitality.

This cookbook isn't just a collection of recipes; it's a testament to the power of plant-based nutrition in managing and even thriving with type 2 diabetes. By embracing a diet rich in protein from sources like legumes, tofu, tempeh, and nuts, we've discovered a flavorful and satisfying way to support our health goals while enjoying every bite.

From energizing breakfasts to hearty dinners, from satisfying snacks to indulgent desserts, each recipe has been crafted with care to nourish both body and soul. But beyond the kitchen, this book serves as a roadmap for a lifestyle rooted in balance, mindfulness, and self-care.

As we embark on our culinary adventures armed with the knowledge and recipes found here, let us remember that every meal is an opportunity to nurture ourselves and cultivate health. Whether we're cooking for ourselves, our families, or our friends, let us approach each dish with intention, gratitude, and joy.

May this book inspire you to explore the endless possibilities of plant-based cooking, to savor the flavors of wholesome ingredients, and to embrace the journey toward better health with open arms and an open heart. Here's to delicious meals, vibrant health, and a future filled with vitality. Bon appétit!

www.ingramcontent.com/pod-product-compliance
Lightning Source LLC
Chambersburg PA
CBHW071027250726
48653CB00005B/1740